YOUR KNOWLEDGE HAS VALUE

The Role of Think Tanks in Combatting COVID-19 and Improving Pandemic Preparedness

Ariatani Wolff

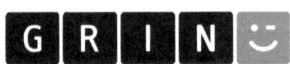

Bibliographic information published by the German National Library:

The German National Library lists this publication in the National Bibliography; detailed bibliographic data are available on the Internet at http://dnb.dnb.de.

ISBN: 9783346851987
This book is also available as an ebook.

Print and binding: Books on Demand GmbH, Norderstedt, Germany
Printed on acid-free paper from responsible sources.

The present work has been carefully prepared. Nevertheless, authors and publishers do not incur liability for the correctness of information, notes, links and advice as well as any printing errors.

GRIN web shop: https://www.grin.com/document/1344166

Table of contents

Introduction

During the COVID-19 pandemic, many actors within the think tanks sector and beyond emphasized that the relevance of research institutions and policy institutes could not be overestimated, which is well illustrated by the following quote from Professor Leach, Director of the *Institute of Development Studies*:

"The COVID-19 pandemic is a health crisis of massive proportions and will have major long-term social, economic and political impacts in countries all over the world. Think tanks globally have an absolutely vital role to play in generating the diverse and collaborative knowledge, action and leadership needed to bring an end to the outbreak and build back more equitable and sustainable societies."
Melissa Leach (qtd. fr. Think Tanks and Civil Societies Program (TTCSP) and The Lauder Institute at the University of Pennsylvania 2020: 18)

Like never before, think tanks had to measure up to their self-claim to provide independent, high-quality research and practical policy recommendations. At the same time, they were confronted with challenges many institutions and companies that used to rely on analogue work faced during the pandemic, among others increased stress and worries of their staff followed by decreasing productivity. For think tanks this problem was accompanied by a serious lack of new research funding as a study from *On Think Tanks (OTT)* about the COVID-19 impacts on the sector found (cf. Mendizabal 2020). However, the same study showed that the respondents (from whom nearly 85 % worked either for a think tank or a policy research programme or department) were relatively optimistic regarding the pandemic effects on their research institutions. Only 16,4 % reported serious concern about the future of their institution whereas 44 % expected to be challenged but able to handle the situation well. 31 % did not even expect too many disrupting changes because their institutes had already established remote work before (idem. 6). Some answers even had a positive angle, as the study participants expected a modernisation towards digitalization, an expansion of their potential audience due to the establishment of webinars, and the development of new decentralized, agile work methods (idem. 7f.).

In line with these ambitious attempts to adapt to the new circumstances, many think tanks managed to continue with their research and used their resources to support the global fight against the pandemic. To show **in which way they have influenced the handling of the pandemic and which policy recommendations they did provide to improve pandemic preparedness** is the key purpose of this paper.

Its main part starts with a definition of the elusive term ‚think tank' to set the scene for the following examination.
To then get a better understanding of their role during the pandemic, the activities of the think tank sector will be exemplified by focusing on two relevant think tanks that will be introduced afterwards, namely the *Center for Strategic and International Studies (CSIS)* and the *European Council on Foreign Relations (ECFR)*.
This section is followed by the discussion of their research and advice as well as their relationship to other (international) institutions that were concerned with the fight against COVID-19.
Afterwards, the future of health systems and health care is discussed in order to identify potential developments and challenges such as the risk that further pandemics will emerge.

To examine the influence think tanks could have on improving the prevention and containment of such incidents, their recommendations regarding pandemic preparedness and necessary health care reforms are presented, focusing once again on the two exemplary think tanks. The conclusion will review the key question and discuss some possible approaches for further research about the role of scientific advice from think tanks during health emergencies.

Main part

Definition of the term ‚think tank'

A uniform definition of the term ‚think tank' does not exist, however, most explanations are well summarized by the characteristics listed in the *Merriam-Webster Dictionary* that describes a think tank as "an institute, corporation, or group organized to study a particular subject (such as a policy issue or a scientific problem) and provide information, ideas, and advice" (Merriam-Webster Dictionary 2022). The platform *TechTarget* provides a corresponding, but more detailed definition: "A think tank is an organization that gathers a group of interdisciplinary scholars to perform research around particular policies, issues, or ideas. Topics addressed in think tanks can cover a wide range, including social policy, public policy, economic policy, political strategy, culture and technology. Think tanks can also be referred to as think factories or policy institutes." (Lewis 2022) Overall, the work of these institutions could be summarized with activities such as "conducting scholarly research, creating a space for debate, generating ideas, monitoring public policy and providing intellectual resources to the public." (Idem.)

The *Think Tank and Civil Societies Program (TTCSP)* conducts research about challenges and trends think tanks as well as policymakers and policy-oriented groups within the civil society are concerned with. This institution often referred to as ‚think tank for think tanks' aims to support regional, national, and global think tanks with advice and resources, enabling them to serve policymakers and the public even better (cf. Think Tanks and Civil Societies Program (TTCSP) and The Lauder Institute at the University of Pennsylvania 2020: 2). Maintaining and relying on a database of over 8,000 think tanks around the world, it explains their structure and role within the political sphere and society as follows: "Think tanks may be affiliated or independent institutions that are structured as permanent bodies, not ad-hoc commissions. These institutions often act as a bridge between the academic and policymaking communities and between states and civil society, serving in the public interest as an independent voice that translates applied and basic research into a language that is understandable, reliable and accessible for policymakers and the public" (McGann 2021a: 13).

According to the "2020 Go To Think Tank Report" published by the *TTCSP*, at least 11,175 think tanks existed in 2020, with the majority based in the USA (2,203), followed by China (1,413) and – by a wide margin – India (612) and the United Kingdom (515) (idem. 43f.). More than half of them were established after 1980 since their rise was promoted by the globalization, the increasing complexity of international challenges, and the end of the Cold War. Another development is that emerging countries especially in Asia have started to catch up, however, the US still has the greatest number of well-established think tanks (cf. McGann 2021b: 187). Think tanks differ significantly in their size, research focus, and in terms of their funding sources, with some being autonomous and independent whereas others are affiliated to universities, governments, political parties or companies (cf. McGann 2021a: 13f.).

Introduction of two exemplary think tanks: *CSIS* and *ECFR*

The two examples were chosen since both are established, international known think tanks that cover a wide range of topics and occupy high ranks in several *TTCSP* think tank rankings such as the "2020 Top Global Health Policy Think Tanks" (McGann 2021a: 179) and the "2020 Think Tanks with the Most Innovative Policy Ideas/Proposals" (idem. 308f.) that are relevant for the key question of this paper. As they have their headquarters in Ottawa (*CSIS*) respectively in seven European capitals (*ECFR*), they do have a regional focus on the US and Europe but also deal with international topics affecting and concerning these states. Due to their size and position within the community of research institutions they managed to adapt quickly to the new working conditions under the COVID-19 pandemic. Because of that and their relatively stable funding situation, they were able to continue with their research whereas especially policy think tanks in developing countries experienced the pandemic as much greater disruption that even questioned the existence of some (cf. e.g. Babu 2020).

In addition to the general definition provided above, the self-descriptions and purposes of the *CSIS* and the *ECFR* are relevant to understand how they see their own work and to examine the extent to which they were able to live up to the role they wanted to play in the fight against COVID-19 and its consequences.

The 1962 founded *CSIS* describes itself as "a bipartisan, nonprofit policy research organization dedicated to advancing practical ideas to address the world's greatest challenges" (CSIS 2022a) to which the COVID-19 pandemic undoubtedly belonged to. Its purpose is "to define the future of national security" (idem.), whereby the term ‚security' is widely defined and also includes the health of the US population. Due to its own values, the think tank claims to be non-partisan, independent, integer, and cross-disciplinary. Moreover, it has the goal to not only conduct high-quality research but also to provide policy recommendations that shape decision-making processes and have noticeable positive effects (cf. idem.).
To do so, the *CSIS* could dispose of $42,8 million in 2019 of which most came from corporate grants and distributions (30 %), foundation grants (29 %), and the US government (24 %). This money was spent completely to finance its different programs (70 %), to cover management and additional costs, and to invest in development (6 %), adding up to $42,9 million of expenses in 2019 (CSIS 2022b).

The *ECFR* describes itself as an "international think-tank that aims to conduct cutting-edge independent research on European foreign and security policy and to provide a safe meeting space for decision-makers, activists and influencers to share ideas." (ECFR 2022) In order to do so the think tank aims to "build coalitions for change at the European level and promote informed debate about Europe's role in the world." (Idem.) Founded in 2007, the *ECFR* is the only think tank with a clear pan-European profile, and gives scholars, national political decision-makers, ambassadors, business as well as civil society leaders, European commissioners, and journalists a forum to discuss the most pressing political challenges, bringing in their different national perspectives and expert knowledge to develop ideas for a common European foreign policy.

As independent, non-profit organization, the *ECFR* is mostly funded by donations, legacies, and charitable activities that added up to total incoming resources of 8,3 € million in 2019. The biggest part of the expenditures of 7,7 € million were spent to finance its five different research programs that deal with Asia, Africa, the Middle East and North Africa, wider Europe, and European Power (cf. ECFR 2020).

As these self-descriptions show, the overall goal of both think tanks goes along with the position of the *TTCSP* that described the common mission of think tanks in a 2021 report as "helping to bridge the gap between knowledge and policy" (McGann et al. 2021: 3).

Role of think tanks during the COVID-19 pandemic

When Sars-Cov-2 began to spread in early 2020, it was the *TTCSP* that initiated a prompt reaction of the global think tank community by organizing an international conference on April 7, 2020. This meeting was the first of three so-called *Global Think Tank Town Halls* under the motto ‚Saving Lives and Livelihood' that brought together several hundred participants who represented think tanks, governments, international organizations (IOs), and non-governmental organizations (NGOs) from 94 different countries (cf. McGann et al. 2021: 5–8). The purpose was to stand in solidarity with those who were hit hardest by the pandemic but was not limited to this demonstration of unity. Instead, five working groups were established that should develop programs and policy advice to support the common fight against COVID-19. Each group focused on a different pandemic-related challenge: The first group developed and discussed strategies how the public health crisis could be addressed effectively; the second focused on international and national strategies to accelerate the economic recovery and revitalization; the third identified innovative, inclusive, public and private strategies to support the most vulnerable social groups; the forth discussed how multilateral, rapid, responsive, and resilient systems could be created to be better prepared for future crises, and the last group developed new operating models for think tanks, re-thinking their traditional way to conduct research, communicate and obtain funding (cf. McGann 2021a: 19–21).

At the second *Global Town Hall* in May 2020, their first results and findings were discussed, looking both at challenges for think tanks itself and at ways how they could promote the crisis management and decision-making processes of their national governments in the changed environment. Moreover, the participants of each group worked on the next sub goal which was the finalization of an action-oriented report including concrete policy recommendations by the beginning of the third and final *Town Hall* (cf. McGann et al. 2021: 5).

When this last conference took place on June 30, 2020, the five reports were presented, discussed, and summarized before the compiled results were conveyed to national governments, the *G20* and the *G7* as well as to relevant IOs and NGOs (idem.).

Although this common approach had some potential, it received too little attention outside the think tank community which means that the target of its initiators to "bridge the gap between knowledge and policy" (McGann et al. 2021: 3) could not be fully met. Although the pandemic was obviously a global challenge which could be only overcome by an international effort, the approach of the *Global Think Tank Town Halls* was probably too academic and produced advice that was unsuitable to be practically implemented on a national level.

Nevertheless, think tanks *did* play a vital role by generating knowledge about the pandemic and its consequences, but their advice had a greater impact when it was precisely directed to single decision-making bodies like national governments or institutions within the international health system. By considering their possible scope of action more targeted advice was given, for example practical steps that could be integrated in the strategies of national governments to combat the pandemic (see McGann 2021: 9ff. for examples). Because of that, the next chapter takes a more detailed look at the two institutions used as examples to understand the role individual think tank advice played for the development of COVID-19 responses.

Research and policy advice of think tanks during the pandemic: Focus on *CSIS* and *ECFR*

As the following table shows, think tanks from all world regions have published pandemic-related reports, launched new research programs or established commissions to provide political advice how to address the global health crisis (cf. Table 1).

Overall, those projects matched their general local and thematic orientation and was therefore often not directly related to the health dimension of COVID-19 but focused on the impact the pandemic had on the focus topics of the single think tanks. The Israelian *Institute for National Security Studies (INSS),* for example, launched a new research program that focused on the nexus between national security, pandemics and climate change (cf. INSS 2023). In distinction to this, the *Menassat for Research and Social Studies* is more interested in the social circumstances within a country than in its security situation and therefore conducted a highly regarded study that aimed to understand how the Moroccan population viewed the challenges posed by the COVID-19-pandemic (cf. Mechouat et al. 2020).

Think tank	Projects & reports to provide policy advice during the pandemic	Country
Center for Strategic and International Studies (CSIS)	Commission: "The CSIS Commission on Strengthening America's Health Security" (2018)	USA
Heritage Foundation	Commission: "National Coronavirus Recovery Commission" (2020)	USA
The Stimson Center	Report: "Coping with New and Old Crises: Global and Regional Cooperation in an Age of Epidemic Uncertainty" (December 2020)	USA
Center for International Governance Innovation (CIGI)	Report: "Re-Imagining a Canadian National Security Strategy for the 21st Century" (2021)	Canada
European Council on Foreign Relations (ECFR)	Policy Brief: "Health sovereignty: How to build a resilient European response to pandemics" (June 2020)	EU
The Royal Institute of International Affairs (Chatham House)	Advisory body: "COVAX Manufacturing Task Force" (March 2020)	UK
LSE IDEAS	Digital platform: "Better together" (April 2020) Conference: "Lessons of the Territorial Peace in Times of COVID-19" (November 2020)	UK
EdLab Asia	Study: "Toward Sustainable Learning during School Suspension: Socioeconomic, Occupational Aspirations, and Learning Behavior of Vietnamese Students during COVID-19" (2020)	Vietnam
Institute for National Security Studies (INSS)	Research program: "Climate Change, Pandemics, and National Security" (September 2020)	Israel
TRENDS Research & Advisory	Book: "The Road to Success, UAE Model in Confronting Covid-19" (April 2020)	UAE
Arab Forum for Alternatives	Study: "COVID-19 Pandemic: Does the Mainstream Public Policies System Achieve Protection for All?" (2020)	Egypt
Menassat For Research and Social Studies	Study: "Moroccans and Covid-19: Representations, attitudes and practices" (July 2020)	Morocco
Centro de Pensamiento Estratégico Internacional (CEPEI)	Centre: "Covid-19 Data and Innovation Centre" (December 2020)	Argentina
Brazilian Center for International Relations (CEBRI)	Report: "Brazil-China Post-Covid-19: Food Security, Food Safety and Sustainability" (2020)	Brazil

Table 1: Exemplary compilation of relevant think tanks and their pandemic-related projects and reports (own presentation according to TTCSP 2020: 10–13, 16–18, 23–25, 27, 31, 34f., 55).

This observation also applies to the *CSIS* and *ECFR*, which should be considered in more detail.

The *CSIS Commission on Strengthening America's Health Security* was first established in 2018 and concerned with multiple projects regarding the health situation of the US population before the COVID-19 pandemic hit the USA. Especially during the first months of 2020 that were characterized by a lack of data and information about the new virus, the government benefitted from the Commission's research as many recommendations could be adjusted to combat the new health crisis. Its members and experts permanently reviewed and workshopped their advice which was then integrated into the plan of the Biden administration to fight the pandemic (cf. CSIS Commission on Strengthening America's Health Security 2022). A good example for the output of this work is the paper "2022 is the Year of Decision" (Brooks et al. 2022) that was published in January 2022 and contains both learnings derived from the past pandemic experiences and recommendations for the future containment strategy. The Commission summarized the learnings from 2021 in ten statements, explaining the most important shortcomings in the strategy of national and international decision-makers to contain the spread of the coronavirus. This inventory was followed by eight very specific pieces of advice to the US government. Starting with the proposal to launch a "US global pandemic initiative" (idem. 3) over demanding more (financial) support for international organizations such as the Coalition for *Epidemic Preparedness Innovations (CEPI)* up to the advice to strive – despite all ideological, economical and miliary differences and rivalries with China – for closer cooperation on health issues, their recommendations were directed at various areas influenced by the pandemic (idem. 15–20).

With their accurate analysis and their clear statements regarding the leading role the USA should play in the global pandemic response, they combine the claim to not remain in the academic world of research but influence actual political decisions and help to shape the US security strategy.

As the *ECFR* has a clear regional focus on Europe, its COVID-19-related research mostly dealt with the handling of the pandemic by single member states of the *European Union (EU)* as well as its common approaches like the joint vaccine procurement strategy and its consequences on the political landscape of Europe (cf. e.g. Dennison and Puglierin 2021). The think tank published reports and practical advice such as the policy brief "Health sovereignty: How to build a resilient European response to pandemics" (Hackenbroich et al. 2020). The authors conclusively presented how the pandemic has exposed and exacerbated already existing problems, such as the lack of health care workers in many member states, the dependance on goods from countries outside the *EU*, and the slowness of its decision-making processes when rapid and decisive crisis management was needed (cf. idem. 12–17). By comparing six big *EU* member states in detail, the paper identifies the similarities and differences in their health care systems and approaches to contain the pandemic, and shows the deep divide among the *EU* countries regarding their ability to deal with major health emergencies. Accordingly, the authors conclude, the willingness for greater cooperation and solidarity varies greatly as its costs and benefits would be very unevenly distributed (cf. idem. 9–11). Because of that, their recommended actions and strategies focused on the common goals of the *EU*, such as the protection of the single market, key European industries, and supply chains in the face of crises (cf. idem. 22–24, 26f. 27–29).

Overall, the policy brief provides concrete steps how Europe could improve and protect its health sovereignty and shows how this would benefit not only the health care sector but many others as well (cf. idem 30f.). Similar to the aspiration of the *CSIS*, the *ECFR* also wants its suggested roadmap to influence and support the decision-making process of their respective policymakers.

Relationship of think tanks to other institutions in the fight against COVID-19

The previous chapter showed exemplary how think tanks managed to stay relevant for the political decision-making process although they could not provide high quality *medical* advice as this was not their primary task. Instead, the national disease control agencies – such as the *Centers for Disease Control and Prevention (CDC)* in the USA or the German *Robert Koch-Institut (RKI)* – and international institutions, first and foremost the *World Health Organization (WHO)*, were responsible to monitor the course of the pandemic closely, constantly collecting data and organizing the use of medical resources to contain the further spread.

However, think tanks often interacted and cooperated with those national and international organizations and initiatives that were primarily concerned with the health dimension of COVID-19 to share their knowledge and insights with them. By relying on cross-disciplinary approaches, experts with different backgrounds could bring in their perspectives on pandemic-related topics which allowed them to develop solutions that would not only work for one but several sectors. It was important, for example, to also think about the impact on the economy when discussing contact restrictions and curfews, or to consider how economic aids and special rules for some groups would affect the social peace within the society.

Such interactions were also common before the start of the COVID-19 pandemic for which the *Strategic and Technical Advisory Group on Infectious Hazards with Pandemic and Epidemic Potential (STAG-IH)* is a good example. The establishment of this expert group in 2018 can be seen as a learning experience of the Ebola outbreaks in several African countries in the early 2000s and was initiated by the *WHO* for which it is the main advisory body when it comes to global health threats posed by infectious diseases (cf. WHO 2022).

However, the way the *WHO* handled the outbreak of the corona virus showed that the existing bodies were not sufficient to deal with such a major health emergency which was not necessarily due to a lack of knowledge but more to an inadequate implementation: Insights and recommendations of the *STAG-IH* and other experts, including relevant think tanks, often remained unnoticed or could not be implemented in the strategic fight against COVID-19 as funding, staff, and competencies were missing. Of course, there was also a lack of data and information on the virus, especially during the first few months of the pandemic, but many scholars agree that not only national governments but also the *WHO* was inadequately prepared for this challenge (cf. e.g. Bollyky and Patrick 2020, IPPPR 2021). Because of that, in May 2022 the *WHO* governing board reacted to the criticism and decided to form a new *Standing Committee on Health Emergency Prevention, Preparedness and Response* that will be able to meet and act much faster when the director-general of the *WHO* would announce a ,Public Health Emergency of International Concern' in the future (cf. VOA News 2022).

As dramatic as the consequences of the pandemic were, they did show the absolute necessity of international cooperation on health issues and could therefore promote some fundamental changes in the global health network. One example are the current considerations to transform *COVAX,* short for *COVID-19 Vaccines Global Access,* into a permanent mechanism to coordinate the fair distribution of vaccines, medication, and other health goods to all countries in need. Although the international initiative established in April 2020 did not fully meet its goal to ensure the fair and fast distribution of the limited amount of available COVID-19 vaccines among *all* countries by avoiding corruption, inefficiencies, and waste of resources, it was an important instrument to give poor states access to the lifesaving vaccines (cf. e.g.

Berkley 2021, Eccleston-Turner and Upton 2021). The initiative had some weaknesses but a reflection and reform process, guided by medical experts, think tanks concerned with international cooperation, and decision-makers within the global health system, could lead to their elimination and make *COVAX* an important instrument to better prevent and combat future pandemics (cf. e.g. Ducharme 2021, Cioaric et al. 2022).

Research and policy advice from think tanks to improve pandemic preparedness: Focus on *CSIS* and *ECFR*

Before the COVID-19 pandemic started, research and policy advice related to health issues did not belong to the traditional focus areas of most think tanks. However, there were several reports about transformative technologies, health security risks, and biological and chemical weapons from renowned institutions, for example the *Federation of American Scientists* (cf. Bidwell and Bhatt 2016) and the *National Academies of Sciences, Engineering, and Medicine (NASEM)* (cf. NASEM 2018). The think tanks this paper focuses on also worked on those topics for which the *CSIS* report "The U.S. Department of Defense's Role in Health Security: Current Capabilities and Recommendations for the Future" (Morrison and Cullison 2019) and the *ECFR* publication on possible Britain reactions to the use of chemical weapons in Syria are two examples (cf. Blunt and Mercer 2017).
A second group of health-related think tank paper indeed dealt with pandemic preparedness, among others a report from the *Johns Hopkins Center for Health Security (CHS)* about its pandemic tabletop exercise (cf. CHS 2018), and the report of the *Global Preparedness Monitoring Board (GPMB)* regarding the world's ability to prevent a major health threat on a global level (cf. GPMB 2019). However, the far-seeing recommendations of these research institutions had hardly caused any political reactions before Sars-Cov-2 occurred which is why many countries were insufficiently prepared to a health emergency such as the Corona pandemic.

If national governments have something learned from the experiences of the past two years will only become completely evident when the next serious health emergency will occur which is due to many scholars merely a matter of time (cf. e.g. Kuhn and Margellos 2022: 206). In any case, there is no shortage of knowledge and possible strategies how to increase pandemic preparedness as many think tanks have given advice to national governments and international institutions, for example the US-based *National Biodefense Science Board (NBSB)* (cf. NBSB 2021), the international *G20 High Level Independent Panel on Financing the Global Commons for Pandemic Preparedness and Response (HLIP)* (cf. Shanmugaratnam et al. 2021) and also the two think tanks this paper focuses on.

In its policy brief "Health of Nations: How Europe can fight future pandemics" (Dworkin 2022), the *ECFR* published its findings how the European health care system could become more resilient. All recommendations had the common core that the *EU* should actively promote the international cooperation and communication about health care issues whereby it would be particularly important to avoid a purely US-European focus but integrate the perspectives and concerns of different world regions. According to the *ECFR*, the *African Union (AU)* plays a key role as Africa has an enormous need for vaccines and medication, and at the same time a large, as yet unused potential for their production. Because of that, the *EU* should closely cooperate with the *AU* and promote the transfer of European pharmaceutical knowledge and technology to the African continent. Another practical measure to enhance pandemic preparedness would be the establishment of a new permanent *WHO* fund that would be overseen by a representative group of (changing) countries and could be used to tackle health emergencies around the globe faster and more efficiently. Moreover, the *ECFR* recommended that national governments should enhance the surveillance and reporting of potential infectious diseases, provide better funding of their health care systems and work towards greater equity regarding the allocation of countermeasures to fight diseases by recording such agreements in a new international compact on pandemic prevention and control. To tackle not only the omissions of states during the pandemic but also of the *WHO*, the *EU* should promote reforms that would improve the independence, competences, and capacities of the most important international organization on health care (cf. idem.13–16).

The *CSIS* produced a short commentary that summarizes its 2020 findings on how pandemic preparedness should be improved and conveyed those recommendations to the *Independent Panel on Pandemic Preparedness and Response (IPPPR)* (cf. Morrison and Reynolds 2020). The establishment of the panel was a response to one of the resolutions that was adopted by the *73ʳᵈ World Health Assembly* in May 2020. It started its work in September of the same year, aiming to learn from the problems and blind spots COVID-19 revealed, and focusing on the development of new strategies how the capacity for global pandemic prevention, preparedness, and response could be improved (cf. IPPPR 2022).

The advice provided by the *CSIS* has much in common with the *ECFR* recommendations, however, the American think tank put a greater focus on the security dimension of the pandemic in terms of the competition between the major military and economic powers of the world. As their response to COVID-19 was politicized and vaccine diplomacy occurred as a widespread phenomenon, it would be important to "Kickstart High Level Political Leadership" (Morrison and Reynolds 2020) in order to close the "Diplomatic Void" (idem.). Another area the *CSIS* addressed more intensively was the fight against disinformation and conspiracy theories, and the consolidation of the progress that have been made in research about and development of COVID-19 vaccines, medication, and therapies. Moreover, the *CSIS* strongly recommended to invest in preparedness, finally complying with the existing international frameworks on global health such as the binding *International Health Regulations (IHR)*, the *Joint External Evaluations (JEE)*, and the *Global Health Security Agenda 2024 Framework* whose implementation has been assured by more than 70 states. Similar to the *ECFR*, the *CSIS* recommended the establishment of a fonds indented for the fight against global health security challenges that would be both publicly and privately financed but independent from national governments. Another similarity was the urgent request to promote *WHO* reforms, enhancing the inspection power and global surveillance capacities of the organization. While the *ECFR* recommended a new pandemic compact, the *CSIS* proposed a global summit in which national head of states should made binding commitments in response to the recommendations presented by the *IPPPR*. In summary, only long-term investments, effective *WHO* reforms, a strict demarcation from anti-science forces, and the commitment to international cooperation could lead to global health system that would be better prepared for future pandemics (cf. idem.).

Overall, these think tank papers on pandemic preparedness show the same aspiration as their advice during the COVID-19 pandemic since they have a clear practical focus and aim to not only inform an educated readership but shape the decision-making process of political leaders and international bodies.

The future of health systems, health care, and the role of think tanks in the global health system

The experience of COVID-19 has changed the global health system and is likely to have serious long-lasting consequences although their scope cannot be fully estimated yet.

One example for negative impacts is the noticeable increase of depressive disorders during the last two years which still challenges many national health care systems as they suffer from a lack of professional therapists and treatment services. In some business sectors, the pandemic caused mass dismissals that led to financial concerns of then unemployed people. Many self-employed people as well as gastronomy operators, artists, and other workers whose jobs were reliant on personal meetings and services were even confronted with insolvency concerns, and could save their businesses only by resorting to financial aid programs (cf. e.g. OECD 2020). Moreover, several studies identified a relationship between COVID-19 lockdowns and increased domestic violence, for example a report from the *National Commission on Covid-19 and Criminal Justice* launched by the *Council on Criminal Justice (CCJ)* according to which domestic violence in the US increased by 8.1 % after the government implemented lockdown orders during the first waves of the pandemic in 2020 (cf. e.g. Piquero et al. 2021). Suffering from loneliness and the fact that people could not meet their loved ones, even when they were ill or dying, are other exemplary factors that were shown to have a negative impact on the public (mental) health situation which was expressed in rising numbers of people suffering from anxiety, depressions, and other mental illnesses (cf. e.g. Ernst et al. 2022, Allen et al. 2022). To make matters worse, the shortage of therapists and treatment options mentioned above was even reinforced as ‚essential workers' – such as employees within the health care sector – were even more likely to be affected by those diseases themselves (cf. Panchal et al. 2021).

As another consequence of the new living and working conditions due to COVID-19, the adoption of digital technologies was accelerated in multiple areas. But not only political negotiations and business meetings were moved to online video meeting platforms, also doctor's appointments that did not urgently require the presence of the patient took place online, and the health tech sector experienced a significant upturn (cf. e.g. Think Tank of the European Parliament 2021). In addition to that, the pandemic promoted the digital collection and exchange of health-related data. As scholars found that countries which already had a digital health infrastructure and managed to quickly and effectively establish additional telemedicine services were able to fight the health crises better (cf. e.g. Fagherazzi et al. 2020, Olesch 2020), governments will probably integrate higher health tech investments into their strategies to strengthen their health care systems and improve their national preparedness for similar future emergencies.

This is without any doubt absolutely necessary as there is a great consensus within the research community that it is only a matter of time when the next dangerous virus will emerge and spread (cf. e.g. Dulaney 2020, Kuhn and Margellos 2022: 206). How national governments and international institutions will use the meantime to prepare for this incident will decide whether humanity will experience another deathly pandemic, or will be able to fight new viruses or variants more effectively and timely. The research and advice of think tanks around the world can play an important role in this preparation and prevention process, as they consider learnings from the COVID-19 experience and develop better crises responses for the future. However, to benefit from their knowledge it is necessary that their visibility increases even more, and that parliaments, governments, and other decision-makers put a new priority on scientific insights and practical advice on health issues. At some point during the pandemic, the main problem was no longer a lack of knowledge about the characteristics of the virus but differing opinions among policymakers how to interpret this information and find the best policy responses (cf. e.g. Nilsen et al. 2020, Schmelz 2021). Moreover, governments were confronted with practical difficulties in the implementation of their measures to contain its spread which is also an area where think tanks could provide helpful advice (cf. e.g. Maqbool and Khan 2020).

Conclusion

Review of the key question

This paper estimated **the way in which think tanks have influenced the handling of the pandemic, including the policy recommendations they provided during the pandemic and the (still ongoing) evaluation process how to improve pandemic preparedness.** Statements of think tank representatives and participants of the *Global Think Tank Town Halls* in early 2020 show that members of the think tank community may have overestimated their practical influence on COVID-19 related policies. As the pandemic unfolded, it became clear that national governments tended to focus on the interests of their own countries, ignoring the advice of many think tanks and other international institutions that emphasized the importance of multilateralism and cooperation. Although think tanks conducted helpful research, many of their insights remained in their ‚expert bubble' without finding the international attention they deserved.

However, it seemed as their advice got more attention on a national and regional level since it was closely directed to the individual situation of the country and easier to implement in the containment strategy as fewer decision-making bodies were involved. This could be seen, for example, by the case of the *CSIS Commission* whose advice was implemented in the strategy of the Biden administration to combat the pandemic.

Their arguably biggest achievement was not so much their influence in the immediate crisis but in the evaluation process after the big waves of the pandemic subsidized. Closely examining successes, problems, and mistakes, think tanks derived learnings from COVID-19, identified room for improvement, and developed strategies how to better prevent and contain major health emergencies in the future.
A good example is the role the *CSIS* played in establishing the *Financial Intermediary Fund (FIF)* at the *World Bank* in the second half of 2022. The purpose of this institution also known as *The Pandemic Fund* is to finance "critical investments to strengthen pandemic prevention, preparedness, and response capacities at national, regional, and global levels, with a focus on low- and middle-income countries." (World Bank 2023) As early as fall 2019, the *CSIS Commission* had called on the US government to take the global lead in addressing health risks and advocate for the establishment of a so-called "Pandemic Preparedness Challenge Fund" (CISI Commission on Strengthening America's Health Security 2019) at the *World Bank*. Back then, their proposal faded away but as the COVID-19 pandemic unfolded, it attracted strong support of the Biden administration and within both Congress parties. Moreover, the idea was also accepted on an international level, as the *IPPPR* and the *G20 HLIP* picked it up and

endorsed it in 2021. After the White House defined the establishment of the fund as one of the primary targets on the *Global COVID-10 Summit* in September 2021, the US government led an international advocacy campaign to convince the critics among state leaders and actors within the global health system who were afraid that such a fund could weaken the role of the *WHO* by taking away the financial support of the important funds that already existed (such as the *Global Fund to Fight AIDS, Tuberculosis and Malaria,* for example). This diplomatic offensive contributed significantly to winning the necessary support of decision-makers, first of all the *WHO* director general Ghebreyesus, the president of the *European Commission (EC)* von der Leyen, the Indonesian President Widodo whose country presided over the *G20* at this time, and the South African president Ramaphosa (cf. Reynolds and Morrison 2022). Since the finance ministers and central bank governors of the *G20* agreed on the establishment of the fund too, the first funding round took place at the second *Global COVID-19 Summit* in May 2022 before it was finally endorsed by the *World Bank* in June and launched in November (cf. World Bank 2022).

This project to improve the global pandemic preparedness required the support of many powerful international actors – in the end the financial pledges came from countries such as the USA, Singapore, and Germany as well as from the *EC*, the *Gates Foundation* and the *Wellcome Trust* – but was initially brought forward and recommended by the *CSIS*. In my opinion, this shows exemplary the future role think tanks could play in the politicized and complex international system: Whereas they do not have the legitimacy to make political decisions for countries, alliances, or international organizations, they can act as pioneers in the development of new policy ideas. Thanks to their research findings, years of experience and expert knowledge, they may detect developments and risks of great importance earlier than other actors that are more concerned with daily politics. However, this does not mean that their expertise remains in the academic and political world – instead, this example demonstrates the practical influence of think tank advice for the society. I therefore support the analysis of Morillas that think tanks can only stay relevant in today's complex world if they manage the "shift from acting as a link between academia and politics toward fostering a greater connection between politics and society" (Morillas 2021: 62).

Room for further research

This paper gives only a very brief overview of the advice the *CSIS* and the *ECFR* provided during the pandemic. It could be productive to examine in detail how national and international decision-makers have reacted to their advice, possibly including respectively comparing more think tanks from other world regions in the analysis. Moreover, it would be interesting to evaluate in some months whether and how governments and institutions within the (inter-)national health system will have implement the recommendations on pandemic preparedness think tanks have published recently.

In addition to that, the brief presentation of exemplary pieces of policy advice on COVID-19 could be deepened by comparing the approaches of multiple think tanks in detail, choosing a sample from different countries. By identifying similarities and differences in their recommendations how future pandemics could be prevented and contained, the most pressing problems and most promising strategies – as well as their possibly differing perceptions between states – could be described and analyzed.

References

ALLEN, J., DARLINGTON, O., HUGHES, K. and BELLIS, M. A. (2022): The public health impact of loneliness during the COVID-19 pandemic. In: *BMC Public Health,* Nr. 22 (1654), https://doi.org/10.1186/s12889-022-14055-2.

BABU, S. C. [Agrilinks] (2020): *Revitalizing Policy Think Tanks in Developing Countries: COVID-19 Challenges and Opportunities.* Available at: https://agrilinks.org/post/revitalizing-policy-think-tanks-developing-countries-covid-19-challenges-and-opportunities [Accessed: 03.01.2023].

BERKLEY, S. [Gavi] (2021): *No one is safe until everyone is safe.* Available at: https://www.gavi.org/vaccineswork/no-one-safe-until-everyone-safe [Accessed: 28.04.2022].

BIDWELL, C. A. and BHATT, K. (2016): Use of Attribution and Forensic Science in Addressing Biological Weapon Threats. Monterey, CA: Federation of American Scientists.

BLUNT, C. and MERCER, J. [European Council on Foreign Relations (ECFR)] (2017): How Britain should respond to chemical weapons attacks in Syria. Available at: https://ecfr.eu/publication/how_britain_should_respond_to_chemical_weapons_attacks_in_syria_7307/ [Accessed: 14.01.2023].

BOLLYKY, T. J. and PATRICK, S. M. [Council on Foreign Relations (CFR)] (2020): *Improving Pandemic Preparedness: Lessons From COVID-19.* Available at: https://www.cfr.org/report/pandemic-preparedness-lessons-COVID-19/findings/ [Accessed: 01.01.2023].

BROOKS, S. W., GERBERDING, J. L. and MORRISON, J. S. [CSIS Commission on Strengthening America's Health Security] (2022): 2022 Is the Year of Decision. Available at: https://healthsecurity.csis.org/articles/2022-is-the-year-of-decision/ [Accessed: 14.01.2023].

CENTER FOR STRATEGIC AND INTERNATIONAL STUDIES (CSIS) (2022a): *About Us.* Available at: https://www.csis.org/programs/about-us [Accessed: 05.12.2022].

CENTER FOR STRATEGIC AND INTERNATIONAL STUDIES (CSIS) (2022b): *Financial Information.* Available at: https://www.csis.org/programs/about-us/financial-information [Accessed: 30.12.2022].

CIOARIC, L., FRANKE, M. and JOUENNE-PEYRAT, F. [Europäisches Parlament] (2022): *Implementation and Financing of COVAX: Successes, Challenges and Lessons for the Future.* Available at: https://www.europarl.europa.eu/cmsdata/248200/COVAX_briefing.pdf [Accessed: 01.07.2022].

CISI COMMISSION ON STRENGTHENING AMERICA'S HEALTH SECURITY [Center for Strategic and International Studies (CSIS)] (2019): Ending the Cycle of Crisis and Complacency in U.S. Global Health Security. Available at: https://healthsecurity.csis.org/final-report/ [Accessed: 10.01.2023].

CSIS COMMISSION ON STRENGTHENING AMERICA'S HEALTH SECURITY (2022): *About the Commission.* Available at: https://healthsecurity.csis.org/about/ [Accessed: 02.01.2023].

DENNISON, S. and PUGLIERIN, J. [European Council on Foreign Relations (ECFR)] (2021): Crisis of confidence: How Europeans see their place in the world. Available at: https://ecfr.eu/publication/crisis-of-confidence-how-europeans-see-their-place-in-the-world/ [Accessed: 14.01.2023].

DUCHARME, J. [Time] (2021): *COVAX Was a Great Idea, But Is Now 500 Million Doses Short of Its Vaccine Distribution Goals. What Exactly Went Wrong?* Available at: https://time.com/6096172/covax-vaccines-what-went-wrong/ [Accessed: 01.01.2023].

DULANEY, M. [ABS News | Science] (2020): *The next pandemic is coming – and sooner than we think, thanks to changes to the environment.* Available at: https://www.abc.net.au/news/science/2020-06-07/a-matter-of-when-not-if-the-next-pandemic-is-around-the-corner/12313372 [Accessed: 05.01.2023].

DWORKIN, A. [European Council on Foreign Relations (ECFR)] (2022): *Health of Nations: How Europe Can Fight Future Pandemics.* Available at: https://ecfr.eu/publication/health-of-nations-how-europe-can-fight-future-pandemics/ [Accessed: 09.12.2022].

ECCLESTON-TURNER, M. and UPTON, H. (2021): International Collaboration to Ensure Equitable Access to Vaccines for COVID-19: The ACT-Accelerator and the COVAX Facility. In: *The Milbank Quarterly,* 99, 10.1111/1468-0009.12503. P. 426-449.

ERNST, M., NIEDERER, D., WERNER, A. M., J., C. S., MIKTON, C., ONG, A. D., ROSEN, T., BRÄHLER, E. and E. BEUTEL, M. (2022): Loneliness Before and During the COVID-19 Pandemic: A Systematic Review With Meta-Analysis. In: *American Psychologist,* https://doi.org/10.1037/amp0001005. P. 1–18.

EUROPEAN COUNCIL ON FOREIGN RELATIONS (ECFR) (2020): *Report and Financial Statements For the Year Ended 31 December.* Available at: https://register-of-charities.charitycommission.gov.uk/charity-search?p_p_id=uk_gov_ccew_onereg_charitydetails_web_portlet_CharityDetailsPortlet&p_p_lifecycle=2&p_p_state=maximized&p_p_mode=view&p_p_resource_id=%2Faccounts-resource&p_p_cacheability=cacheLevelPage&_uk_gov_ccew_onereg_charitydetails_web_portlet_CharityDetailsPortlet_objectiveId=A10450827&_uk_gov_ccew_onereg_charitydetails_web_portlet_CharityDetailsPortlet_priv_r_p_mvcRenderCommandName=%2Faccounts-and-annual-returns&_uk_gov_ccew_onereg_charitydetails_web_portlet_CharityDetailsPortlet_priv_r_p_organisationNumber=4049916 [Accessed: 30.12.2022].

EUROPEAN COUNCIL ON FOREIGN RELATIONS (ECFR) (2022): *About ECFR.* Available at: https://ecfr.eu/about/ [Accessed: 05.12.2022].

FAGHERAZZI, G., GOETZINGER, C., RASHID, M. A., AGUAYO, G. A. and HUIART, L. (2020): Digital Health Strategies to Fight COVID-19 Worldwide: Challenges, Recommendations, and a Call for Papers. In: *Journal of Medical Internet Research,* Nr. 22 (6), https://doi.org/10.2196/19284.

GLOBAL PREPAREDNESS MONITORING BOARD (GPMB) (2019): A World at Risk. Available at: https://www.gpmb.org/annual-reports/overview/item/2019-a-world-at-risk [Accessed].

HACKENBROICH, J., SHAPIRO, J. and VARMA, T. [European Council on Foreign Relations (ECFR)] (2020): *Health sovereignty: How to build a resilient European response to pandemics.* Available at: https://ecfr.eu/publication/health_sovereignty_how_to_build_a_resilient_european_response_to_pandemics/ [Accessed: 03.01.2023].

INDEPENDENT PANEL FOR PANDEMIC PREPAREDNESS AND RESPONSE (IPPPR) (2021): Covid: Make it the last pandemic. Available at: https://theindependentpanel.org/wp-content/uploads/2021/05/COVID-19-Make-it-the-Last-Pandemic_final.pdf [Accessed].

INDEPENDENT PANEL FOR PANDEMIC PREPAREDNESS AND RESPONSE (IPPPR) (2022): *About the Independent Panel.* Available at: https://theindependentpanel.org/about-the-independent-panel/ [Accessed: 30.12.2022].

INSTITUTE FOR NATIONAL SECURITY STUDIES (INSS) (2023): *Climate Change and National Security*. Available at: https://www.inss.org.il/subjects_tags/climate-change-and-national-security/ [Accessed: 02.01.2023].

JOHNS HOPKINS CENTER FOR HEALTH SECURITY (CHS) (2018): Clade X Excercise: Improving Policy to Prepare for Severe Pandemics.

KUHN, B. M. and MARGELLOS, D. L. (2022): Health and Nutrition. In: Kuhn, B. M. and Margellos, D. L. [ed.]: *Global Perspectives on Megatrends. The Future as Seen by Analysts and Researchers from Different World Regions.* Hannover: ibidem-Verl. P. 193–218.

LEWIS, S. [TechTarget] (2022): *Definition: think tank*. Available at: https://www.techtarget.com/searchcio/definition/think-tank#:~:text=A%20think%20tank%20is%20an,political%20strategy%2C%20culture%20and%20technology. [Accessed: 30.12.2022].

MAQBOOL, A. and KHAN, N. Z. (2020): Analyzing barriers for implementation of public health and social measures to prevent the transmission of COVID-19 disease using DEMATEL method. In: *Diabetes and Metabolic Syndrome: Clinical Research and Reviews,* Nr. 14 (5), https://doi.org/10.1016/j.dsx.2020.06.024. P. 887–892.

MCGANN, J. G. [Think Tanks and Civil Societies Program (TTCSP)] (2021a): 2020 Global Go To Think Tank Index Report. Available at: https://repository.upenn.edu/think_tanks/18 [Accessed].

MCGANN, J. G. (2021b): Global Trends and Transitions in Think Tanks, Politics, and Policy Advice in the Age of Policy Dilemmas and Disruptions. In: Wang, H. and Michie, A. [ed.]: *Consensus or Conflict?. China and Globalizatioon.* Singapore: Springer. P. 179–190.

MCGANN, J. G., NOOR, Z., LACEWALA, A. and MACRI, J. [Think Tanks and Civil Societies Program (TTCSP), University of Pennsylvania] (2021): *Think Tanks & Pandemic Policy Advice (2020-21)*. Available at: https://repository.upenn.edu/ttcsp_papers/9 [Accessed: 09.12.2022].

MECHOUAT, A., RAHOUTI, M., ADOUNI, H. and ET. AL. (2020): Moroccans and Covid-19: Representations, attitudes and practices. Casablanca: Menassat For Research and Social Science.

MENDIZABAL, E. [On Think Tanks (OTT)] (2020): COVID-19 Initiative: Survey Results. Available at: https://onthinktanks.org/wp-content/uploads/2020/07/COVID-19_SurveyReport_1.pdf [Accessed: 07.01.2023].

MERRIAM-WEBSTER DICTIONARY (2022): *Definition: think tank*. Available at: https://www.merriam-webster.com/dictionary/think%20tank [Accessed: 30.12.2022].

MORILLAS, P. (2021): Connecting Politics and Society: AWay Forward for Think Tanks. In: Mcgann, J. [ed.]: *The Future of Think Tanks and Policy Advice Around the World.* Hampshire, UK: Palgrave Macmillan. P. 59–62.

MORRISON, S. J. and CULLISON, T. R. (2019): The U.S. Department of Defense's Role in Health Security: Current Capabilities and Recommendations for the Future. Center for Strategic and International Studies (CSIS).

MORRISON, S. J. and REYNOLDS, C. [Center for Strategic and International Studies (CSIS)] (2020): *Advice to the Independent Panel on Pandemic Preparedness and Response*. Available at: https://www.csis.org/analysis/advice-independent-panel-pandemic-preparedness-and-response [Accessed: 05.12.2022].

NATIONAL ACADEMIES OF SCIENCES, ENGINEERING, AND MEDICINE (NASEM) (2018): Biodefense in the Age of Synthetic Biology. Washington, DC: National Academic Press.

NATIONAL BIODEFENSE SCIENCE BOARD (NBSB) (2021): Filling Critical Gaps: Comprehensive Recommendations for Public Health Preparedness, Response, and

Recovery from the National Biodefense Science Board. Available at:
https://www.phe.gov/Preparedness/legal/boards/nbsb/meetings/Documents/NBSB-Report-Filling-Critical-Gaps-26May2021-508.pdf [Accessed].

NILSEN, P., SEING, I., ERICSSON, C., ANERSEN, O., STEFÁNSDÓTTIR, N. T., TJØRNHØJ-THOMSEN, T., KALLEMOSE, T. and KIRK, J. W. (2020): Implementing social distancing policy measures in the battle against the coronavirus: protocol of a comparative study of Denmark and Sweden. In: *Implementation Science Communications,* Nr. 1 (77), https://doi.org/10.1186/s43058-020-00065-x.

OLESCH, A. [Healthcare IT News] (2020): *Germany benefits from digital health infrastructure during COVID-19 pandemic.* Available at:
https://www.healthcareitnews.com/news/emea/germany-benefits-digital-health-infrastructure-during-covid-19-pandemic [Accessed: 05.01.2023].

ORGANIZATION FOR ECONOMIC CO-OPERATION AND DEVELOPMENT (OECD) (2020): *OECD Policy Responses to Coronavirus (COVID-19): Insolvency and debt overhang following the COVID-19 outbreak: Assessment of risks and policy responses.* Available at: https://www.oecd.org/coronavirus/policy-responses/insolvency-and-debt-overhang-following-the-covid-19-outbreak-assessment-of-risks-and-policy-responses-7806f078/ [Accessed: 05.01.2023].

PANCHAL, N., KAMAL, R., COX FOLLOW, C. and GARFIELD, R. [Kaiser Family Foundation (KFF)] (2021): *The Implications of COVID-19 for Mental Health and Substance Use.* Available at: https://www.kff.org/coronavirus-covid-19/issue-brief/the-implications-of-covid-19-for-mental-health-and-substance-use/ [Accessed: 04.01.2023].

PIQUERO, A. R., JENNINGS, W. G., JEMISON, E., KAUKINEN, C. and KNAUL, F. M. [National Commission on Covid-19 and Criminal Justice] (2021): Domestic Violence During the COVID-19 Pandemic: Evidence from a Systematic Review and Meta-Analysis. Available at: https://counciloncj.org/impact-report-covid-19-and-domestic-violence-trends/ [Accessed].

REYNOLDS, C. and MORRISON, S. J. [Center for Strategic and International Studies (CSIS)] (2022): *Launching A New Pandemic Preparedness Fund: A Crack in the Cycle of Panic and Neglect?* Available at: https://www.csis.org/analysis/launching-new-pandemic-preparedness-fund-crack-cycle-panic-and-neglect [Accessed: 10.01.2023].

SCHMELZ, K. (2021): Enforcement may crowd out voluntary support for COVID-19 policies, especially where trust in government is weak and in a liberal society. In: *National Academy of Sciences.,* Nr. 118 (1), https://doi.org/10.1073/pnas.2016385118.

SHANMUGARATNAM, T., SUMMERS, L., NGOZI OKONJO-IWEALA, N. and ET AL. (2021): A Global Deal for Our Pandemic Age. G20 High Level Independent Panel on Financing the Global Commons for Pandemic Preparedness and Response (HLIP).

THINK TANK OF THE EUROPEAN PARLIAMENT (2021): *The rise of digital health technologies during the pandemic.* Available at:
https://www.europarl.europa.eu/thinktank/en/document/EPRS_BRI(2021)690548 [Accessed: 05.01.2023].

THINK TANKS AND CIVIL SOCIETIES PROGRAM (TTCSP) and THE LAUDER INSTITUTE AT THE UNIVERSITY OF PENNSYLVANIA (2020): *Global Think Tank Town Hall: Saving Lives and Livelihoods.* Available at:
https://lauder.wharton.upenn.edu/wp-content/uploads/2020/04/Global-Think-Tank-Town-Hall-Draft-Report-4.28.pdf [Accessed: 09.12.2022].

VOA NEWS (2022): *New WHO Panel to Speed Up Pandemic Response, Address Shortcomings.* Available at: https://www.voanews.com/a/new-who-panel-to-speed-up-pandemic-response-address-shortcomings/6595997.html [Accessed: 31.12.2022].

WORLD BANK (2022): *G20 hosts Official Launch of The Pandemic Fund*. Available at: https://www.worldbank.org/en/news/press-release/2022/11/12/g20-hosts-official-launch-of-the-pandemic-fund [Accessed: 10.01.2023].

WORLD BANK (2023): *The Pandemic Fund*. Available at: https://www.worldbank.org/en/programs/financial-intermediary-fund-for-pandemic-prevention-preparedness-and-response-ppr-fif [Accessed: 10.01.2023].

WORLD HEALTH ORGANIZATION (WHO) (2022): *Strategic and Technical Advisory Group for Infectious Hazards with Pandemic and Epidemic Potential (STAG-IH) – About Us*. Available at: https://www.who.int/groups/strategic-and-technical-advisory-group-for-infectious-hazards-(stag-ih)/about-us [Accessed: 31.12.2022].

YOUR KNOWLEDGE HAS VALUE

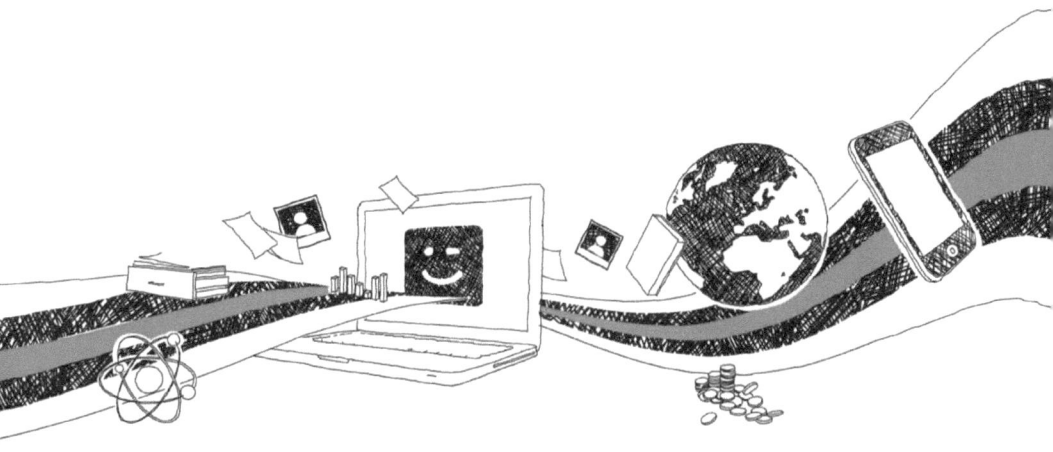

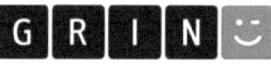